CHAPTER ONE

Introduction to Ibuprofen

Ibuprofen is a commonly used NSAID that was first developed in the 1960s by Dr. Stewart Adams and colleagues at Boots Group. The drug was originally licensed for the treatment of rheumatoid arthritis but very soon became a bestseller because of its relative safety compared to the other NSAIDs, which were used for treating this disease at that time, and its proven efficacy compared with aspirin and indomethacin. Racemic ibuprofen is described chemically as

(RS)-2-(4-(2-methylpropyl)phenyl)propanoic acid. It is a member of the propionic acid class of NSAIDs, possesses a chiral center, and consequently has two enantiomeric forms, S-ibuprofen and R-ibuprofen. The S-enantiomer ex

Ibuprofen is available in various forms: tablets,

capsules, suspensions, gels for topic administration, and IV forms. It is the OTC drug for lower doses and a prescription drug for high doses. This drug is marketed under different brand names, including Advil, Motrin, and Nurofen.

Mechanism of Action

Inhibition of Cyclooxygenase (COX) Enzymes

The principal mode of action for ibuprofen is cyclooxgenase-1 and -2 enzyme inhibition, both COX-1 and COX-2. Cyclooxygenase is an enzyme that drives the process whereby arachidonic acid is turned into prostaglandins.

Prostaglandins are lipids acting as autocrine and paracrine factors that mediate inflammation, pain, and fever.

Ibuprofen inhibits the function of COX enzymes,

reducing prostaglandin synthesis in that regard, and ultimately reduces inflammation, pain, and an increase in body temperature. COX-1 is involved in maintaining normal gastrointestinal and renal functions, while COX-2 is inducible and normally associated with inflammatory processes.

Analgesic Effect; pain is reduced through a decrease in prostaglandin synthesis, which.

Inhibition of prostaglandin synthesis within the hypothalamus reduces fever because it is the central control of the body temperature in the brain.

The anti-inflammatory properties of ibuprofen are due to the inhibition of COX-2. As a consequence, it diminishes the production of pro-inflammatory prostaglandins at the site of inflammation.

Therapeutic Uses

Ibuprofen has widespread use for the relief of many kinds of pain

It is effective against headaches and migraines in reducing the severity and frequency.

It can be used in case of muscle strains, sprains, and

other musculoskeletal injuries.

Ibuprofen also assists in reducing inflammation and pain with regards to osteoarthritis, rheumatoid arthritis, and other types of arthritis.

It minimizes the severity of menstrual cramps by stopping the action of the uterus from producing more prostaglandin. It is commonly given post-dental extraction or due to toothache.

Ibuprofen is a very good febrile agent and can be used to reduce fever in adults and children. It is preferred over many antipyretic agents as it has additional properties against pain.

Ibuprofen can provide inflammation control by decreasing swelling and enhancing function in any pathological condition with massive inflammation, for instance, bursitis, tendinitis, and gout.

Ibuprofen is often used in neonatal units to close the patent ductus arteriosus (PDA) that remains open after birth in some patients, while additional functions of this drug will be described in the following part of the work.

Administration and Dosage

Ibuprofen is available in multiple strengths and formulations, thus making it useful across numerous age groups and conditions. The mainstay of administration should necessarily follow the prescribed dosage and administration guidelines in order to maintain its efficacy for the treatment.

In case of pain and fever, the usual dose for every adult is 200-400 mg orally every 4-6 hours as needed. The maximum dose in 24 hours is 3200 mg.

The dose for chronic ailments, such as arthritis, is 400-800 mg three to four times a day. Dosage adjustments should be done according to the appropriate clinical response and tolerance.

The dose for children will be calculated by body weight. It is usually 10 mg/kg every 6-8 hours. Maximum daily dose is 40 mg/kg.

In preterm infants, ibuprofen is administered intravenously. The dose to be administered is usually based on the weight of the baby and his condition.

Patients with hepatic or renal impairment may have altered drug metabolism and excretion. Thus, this may need a dose adjustment.

A reduced dose may be required in elderly patients because they are increasingly prone to side effects, which may further worsen comorbid conditions in this category of patients.

Administration Tips

It is generally said that taking ibuprofen with food or milk will help reduce gastrointestinal upset.

Patients should not take alcohol while on ibuprofen. It can increase the chance of causing gastrointestinal bleeding.

Adverse Effects

The gastrointestinal adverse effects comprise nausea, vomiting, dyspepsia, and heartburn, whereas, dizziness, headache, and drowsiness are the most common CNS adverse effects, which occur more in higher doses.

Skin rashes and itching are relatively common.

Prolonged use or high doses of ibuprofen may result in gastrointestinal bleeding, ulceration, and perforation.

An increased risk for myocardial infarction, stroke, and hypertension has been associated with its long-term use, especially in people with previous cardiovascular history.

Chronic use of ibuprofen may result in renal impairment or failure, particularly in patients with pre-existing renal disease or those receiving other nephrotoxic drugs.

Anaphylactic reactions, including angioedema and

bronchospasm, may develop, especially in patients allergic to NSAIDs.

Monitoring and Managing Side Effects

Long-term users need their renal and liver function tests monitored.

Gastroprotective drugs like proton pump inhibitors or H2-receptor antagonists can be given concomitantly to reduce the occurrence of possible gastrointestinal side effects.

Patients should be informed about serious side effects that need to be reported urgently, including signs of gastrointestinal bleeding (e.g., black stools, bloody stools) and signs of cardiovascular events (e.g., chest pain, shortness of breath).

CHAPTER TWO

Interactions with Other Drugs

Being a compound that presents with such a property, the combination between them and ibuprofen may result in an increased therapeutic response of anticoagulants like warfarin and antiplatelet agents, such as aspirin.

NSAIDs, including ibuprofen, reduce the antihypertensive effects of ACE inhibitors, angiotensin II receptor blockers (ARBs), and diuretics.

Ibuprofen attenuates the natriuretic effects due to attenuation by reducing the effect of diuretics like furosemide and thiazides and can cause sodium and fluid retention, which eventually causes the exacerbation of heart failure. It is worth knowing that Ibuprofen increases the serum levels and, hence, toxicity of. Methotrexate plasma levels and hence its toxicity can be increased when given concurrently with ibuprofen. The nephrotoxic effects of cyclosporine are exacerbated when administered with ibuprofen.

Prevention of Adverse Interactions

Patients should consult with healthcare providers regarding all other drugs they are taking, including OTC drugs and supplements.

Dose adjustment and tight monitoring can be done with the use of interacting drugs along with ibuprofen.

Contraindications and Precautions

Known hypersensitivity to ibuprofen or other NSAIDs, as manifested by asthma, urticaria, or allergic-type reactions after taking aspirin or other NSAIDs

Patients with current or recent history of

gastrointestinal bleeding or peptic ulcer disease Patients with significant renal or hepatic dysfunction. Ibuprofen is contraindicated during pregnancy's third trimester because it may cause the premature closure of the ductus arteriosus.

Relative Contraindications and Precautions

Ibuprofen is used with extreme caution and strictly under medical supervision in individuals with a history of peptic ulcer disease or gastrointestinal bleeding. High-dose or long-term use of ibuprofen is linked with higher risks of myocardial infarction and stroke among patients with, or at high risk for cardiovascular disease.

Ibuprofen can precipitate bronchospasm in patients with asthma; it should thus be used carefully in this population.

It is to be used cautiously in mild or moderate renal or

hepatic impartment. The renal and hepatic functions should be closely monitored. Dosage adjustments and monitoring need to be close in the elderly because the risk for side effects is more in them.

Ibuprofen compared with other NSAIDs

As an antiplatelet effect, common throughout the world, but risk of the side effect on gastrointestinal is higher compared to ibuprofen.

Naproxenhas the same function as ibuprofen, but

with a longer half-life, so it can be administered less frequently. It may have slight risks of gastrointestinal bleeding.

Celecoxib is an agent that is COX-2 selective, has generally less gastric effect, but more cardiovascular risks.

Ibuprofen, naproxen, and aspirin are effective for mild to moderate pain. The choice of which NSAID is often determined by patient tolerance and specific indications.

All NSAIDs have anti-inflammatory properties, but the effect may vary between patients.

Lifestyle Changes

Regular physical function can help to reduce pain and inflammation, improve cardiovascular health, and enhance overall well-being

An anti-inflammatory diet composed of fresh fruits, vegetables, whole grains, and omega-3 fatty acids helps reduce inflammation and improves health prognosis.

THE END